We Care

Care Conference Template for Skilled Nursing Professionals

By Lauren C. Reynolds

Social Services Director, Skilled Nursing

We Care: Care Conference Template for Skilled Nursing Professionals.

Copywrite December 20, 2022 Lauren C. Reynolds

Inclusive of all versions of this work.

All Rights Reserved.
No part of this book may be reproduced, or stored in a retrieval system, or transmitted in any form or by any means, electronic, mechanical, photocopying, recording or otherwise, without express written permission of the publisher.

The views expressed in these publications are those of the author alone and should not be taken as expert instruction or commands. The reader is responsible for his or her own actions.

Adherence to all applicable laws and regulations including international, federal, state, and local governing professional licensing, business practices, advertising, and all other aspects of doing business in the US or Canada, or any other jurisdictions is the sole responsibility of the purchaser or reader.

Neither the author nor the publisher assumes any responsibility or liability whatsoever on the behalf of the purchaser or the reader of these materials.

Any perceived slight of any individual or organization is purely unintentional.

Care Plan Conference   Date:

To identify goals and establish a discharge plan for your rehabilitation patient.

OR Quarterly care conference for long term care resident.

Patient Name: _____

Staff members in attendance names/positions:

Staff Attending Signatures: _____ _____ _____ _____
_____ _____

Family or Friends/ Support Names:

Nursing Review:

Primary diagnosis/ review of recent hospitalization:

> ➢ Copy of Current Care Plan reviewed and provided to patient.
> ➢ Copy of Current Medication List/ Orders reviewed and provided to patient.
> ➢ Does the patient have medication questions?

Any changes or follow up needed with medications –

Weight, Blood Pressure, Vitals Reviewed -

POLST reviewed, does patient prefer CPR or DNR?

Upcoming appointments and who will transport –

Insurance/ payer source reviewed –

Anticipated length of stay –

Barriers to address:

Goals: (examples – stitches out, follow up orthopedic appointment for weight bearing upgrade, medication date noted for completion of antibiotic, etc.)

Does the patient have any questions for nursing?

Speech Therapy Review:

Results of any cognitive testing such as the MoCA (Montreal Cognitive Assessment) and what the testing means -

Cognitive strengths noted or deficits –

Swallow Assessment Completed and results –

Any issues noted with swallow –

Diet texture currently –

Any goal to upgrade or downgrade diet texture –

Cognition based recommendations for assistance at home –

Self-medication program recommended or will medication management be recommended?

Physical Therapy Review -

Define what therapy is working on with patient and helping with, strengthening lower body, improving gait, reducing fall risk.

Prior level of function –

    Transfer status:

    DME used, ie. Hoyer or Mechanical Life, Front wheeled walker, Wheelchair –

    Level of assistance needed prior at home/in community –

    Level of assistance patient is currently needing, standby assist, contact guard assist, maximum assistance of 2 persons?

    Number of feet patient can ambulate –

    Does patient use an assistive device such as a front wheeled walker to ambulate or do they self-propel their wheelchair?

Will goal be to return patient as close to prior level of function as possible, or will patient have a new baseline level of function?

Occupational Therapy Review:

Define what occupational therapy is working on with patient and helping with, ie. Activities of daily living or ADL's.

Prior level of function –

Amount of assistance needed with lower body dressing –

Amount of assistance needed with upper body dressing –

Self Care level of assist, grooming, personal hygiene –

Level of assistance needed with toileting –

Transfer status –

Any recommended adaptive strategies or equipment to promote optimal functioning?

Recommendation for level of care in community – will increased support be recommended at home or a different setting possibly?

Social Services Review and Discharge Planning:

Discharge Plan:

DME (durable medical equipment) recommended:

Resources and support/caregiver contact info. Given to patient:

Mental Health Services recommended?

Patient accepts or declines mental health interventions: Accepts   Declines

Dental needs:

Vision needs:

Does patient want a Medicaid application and/or help completing?

DPOA established, and if not, does patient need assistance to do so?

Medicare/Insurance Process Reviewed:

Home Health Agency:

Funeral Home selected:

Care Plan Conference   Date:

To identify goals and establish a discharge plan for your rehabilitation patient.

OR Quarterly care conference for long term care resident.

Patient Name: _____

Staff members in attendance names/positions:

Staff Attending Signatures: _____ _____ _____ _____

_____ _____

Family or Friends/ Support Names:

Nursing Review:

Primary diagnosis/ review of recent hospitalization:

- ➢ Copy of Current Care Plan reviewed and provided to patient.
- ➢ Copy of Current Medication List/ Orders reviewed and provided to patient.
- ➢ Does the patient have medication questions?

Any changes or follow up needed with medications –

Weight, Blood Pressure, Vitals Reviewed -

POLST reviewed, does patient prefer CPR or DNR?

Upcoming appointments and who will transport –

Insurance/ payer source reviewed –

Anticipated length of stay –

Barriers to address:

Goals: (examples – stitches out, follow up orthopedic appointment for weight bearing upgrade, medication date noted for completion of antibiotic, etc.)

Does the patient have any questions for nursing?

Speech Therapy Review:

Results of any cognitive testing such as the MoCA (Montreal Cognitive Assessment) and what the testing means -

Cognitive strengths noted or deficits –

Swallow Assessment Completed and results –

Any issues noted with swallow –

Diet texture currently –

Any goal to upgrade or downgrade diet texture –

Cognition based recommendations for assistance at home –

Self-medication program recommended or will medication management be recommended?

Physical Therapy Review -

Define what therapy is working on with patient and helping with, strengthening lower body, improving gait, reducing fall risk.

Prior level of function –

    Transfer status:

    DME used, ie. Hoyer or Mechanical Life, Front wheeled walker, Wheelchair –

    Level of assistance needed prior at home/in community –

Level of assistance patient is currently needing, standby assist, contact guard assist, maximum assistance of 2 persons?

Number of feet patient can ambulate –

Does patient use an assistive device such as a front wheeled walker to ambulate or do they self-propel their wheelchair?

Will goal be to return patient as close to prior level of function as possible, or will patient have a new baseline level of function?

Occupational Therapy Review:

Define what occupational therapy is working on with patient and helping with, ie. Activities of daily living or ADL's.

Prior level of function –

Amount of assistance needed with lower body dressing –

Amount of assistance needed with upper body dressing –

Self Care level of assist, grooming, personal hygiene –

Level of assistance needed with toileting –

Transfer status –

Any recommended adaptive strategies or equipment to promote optimal functioning?

Recommendation for level of care in community – will increased support be recommended at home or a different setting possibly?

Social Services Review and Discharge Planning:

Discharge Plan:

DME (durable medical equipment) recommended:

Resources and support/caregiver contact info. Given to patient:

Mental Health Services recommended?

Patient accepts or declines mental health interventions: Accepts   Declines

Dental needs:

Vision needs:

Does patient want a Medicaid application and/or help completing?

DPOA established, and if not, does patient need assistance to do so?

Medicare/Insurance Process Reviewed:

Home Health Agency:

Funeral Home selected:

Care Plan Conference   Date:

To identify goals and establish a discharge plan for your rehabilitation patient.

OR Quarterly care conference for long term care resident.

Patient Name: _____

Staff members in attendance names/positions:

Staff Attending Signatures: _____ _____ _____ _____
_____ _____

Family or Friends/ Support Names:

Nursing Review:

Primary diagnosis/ review of recent hospitalization:

- Copy of Current Care Plan reviewed and provided to patient.
- Copy of Current Medication List/ Orders reviewed and provided to patient.
- Does the patient have medication questions?

Any changes or follow up needed with medications –

Weight, Blood Pressure, Vitals Reviewed -

POLST reviewed, does patient prefer CPR or DNR?

Upcoming appointments and who will transport –

Insurance/ payer source reviewed –

Anticipated length of stay –

Barriers to address:

Goals: (examples – stitches out, follow up orthopedic appointment for weight bearing upgrade, medication date noted for completion of antibiotic, etc.)

Does the patient have any questions for nursing?

Speech Therapy Review:

Results of any cognitive testing such as the MoCA (Montreal Cognitive Assessment) and what the testing means -

Cognitive strengths noted or deficits –

Swallow Assessment Completed and results –

Any issues noted with swallow –

Diet texture currently –

Any goal to upgrade or downgrade diet texture –

Cognition based recommendations for assistance at home –

Self-medication program recommended or will medication management be recommended?

Physical Therapy Review -

Define what therapy is working on with patient and helping with, strengthening lower body, improving gait, reducing fall risk.

Prior level of function –

Transfer status:

DME used, ie. Hoyer or Mechanical Life, Front wheeled walker, Wheelchair –

Level of assistance needed prior at home/in community –

Level of assistance patient is currently needing, standby assist, contact guard assist, maximum assistance of 2 persons?

Number of feet patient can ambulate –

Does patient use an assistive device such as a front wheeled walker to ambulate or do they self-propel their wheelchair?

Will goal be to return patient as close to prior level of function as possible, or will patient have a new baseline level of function?

Occupational Therapy Review:

Define what occupational therapy is working on with patient and helping with, ie. Activities of daily living or ADL's.

Prior level of function –

Amount of assistance needed with lower body dressing –

Amount of assistance needed with upper body dressing –

Self Care level of assist, grooming, personal hygiene –

Level of assistance needed with toileting –

Transfer status –

Any recommended adaptive strategies or equipment to promote optimal functioning?

Recommendation for level of care in community – will increased support be recommended at home or a different setting possibly?

Social Services Review and Discharge Planning:

Discharge Plan:

DME (durable medical equipment) recommended:

Resources and support/caregiver contact info. Given to patient:

Mental Health Services recommended?

Patient accepts or declines mental health interventions: Accepts   Declines

Dental needs:

Vision needs:

Does patient want a Medicaid application and/or help completing?

DPOA established, and if not, does patient need assistance to do so?

Medicare/Insurance Process Reviewed:

Home Health Agency:

Funeral Home selected:

Care Plan Conference   Date:

To identify goals and establish a discharge plan for your rehabilitation patient.

OR Quarterly care conference for long term care resident.

Patient Name: _____

Staff members in attendance names/positions:

Staff Attending Signatures: _____   _____   _____   _____
_____   _____

Family or Friends/ Support Names:

Nursing Review:

Primary diagnosis/ review of recent hospitalization:

> ➢ Copy of Current Care Plan reviewed and provided to patient.
> ➢ Copy of Current Medication List/ Orders reviewed and provided to patient.
> ➢ Does the patient have medication questions?

Any changes or follow up needed with medications –

Weight, Blood Pressure, Vitals Reviewed -

POLST reviewed, does patient prefer CPR or DNR?

Upcoming appointments and who will transport –

Insurance/ payer source reviewed –

Anticipated length of stay –

Barriers to address:

Goals: (examples – stitches out, follow up orthopedic appointment for weight bearing upgrade, medication date noted for completion of antibiotic, etc.)

Does the patient have any questions for nursing?

Speech Therapy Review:

Results of any cognitive testing such as the MoCA (Montreal Cognitive Assessment) and what the testing means -

Cognitive strengths noted or deficits –

Swallow Assessment Completed and results –

Any issues noted with swallow –

Diet texture currently –

Any goal to upgrade or downgrade diet texture –

Cognition based recommendations for assistance at home –

Self-medication program recommended or will medication management be recommended?

Physical Therapy Review -

Define what therapy is working on with patient and helping with, strengthening lower body, improving gait, reducing fall risk.

Prior level of function –

    Transfer status:

DME used, ie. Hoyer or Mechanical Life, Front wheeled walker, Wheelchair –

    Level of assistance needed prior at home/in community –

    Level of assistance patient is currently needing, standby assist, contact guard assist, maximum assistance of 2 persons?

    Number of feet patient can ambulate –

Does patient use an assistive device such as a front wheeled walker to ambulate or do they self-propel their wheelchair?

    Will goal be to return patient as close to prior level of function as possible, or will patient have a new baseline level of function?

Occupational Therapy Review:

Define what occupational therapy is working on with patient and helping with, ie. Activities of daily living or ADL's.

    Prior level of function –

    Amount of assistance needed with lower body dressing –

Amount of assistance needed with upper body dressing –

Self-Care level of assist, grooming, personal hygiene –

Level of assistance needed with toileting –

Transfer status –

Any recommended adaptive strategies or equipment to promote optimal functioning?

Recommendation for level of care in community – will increased support be recommended at home or a different setting possibly?

Social Services Review and Discharge Planning:

Discharge Plan:

DME (durable medical equipment) recommended:

Resources and support/caregiver contact info. Given to patient:

Mental Health Services recommended?

Patient accepts or declines mental health interventions: Accepts   Declines

Dental needs:

Vision needs:

Does patient want a Medicaid application and/or help completing?

DPOA established, and if not, does patient need assistance to do so?

Medicare/Insurance Process Reviewed:

Home Health Agency:

Funeral Home selected:

Care Plan Conference   Date:

To identify goals and establish a discharge plan for your rehabilitation patient.

OR Quarterly care conference for long term care resident.

Patient Name: _____

Staff members in attendance names/positions:

Staff Attending Signatures: _____ _____ _____ _____
_____ _____

Family or Friends/ Support Names:

Nursing Review:

Primary diagnosis/ review of recent hospitalization:

- ☐ Copy of Current Care Plan reviewed and provided to patient.
- ☐ Copy of Current Medication List/ Orders reviewed and provided to patient.
- ☐ Does the patient have medication questions?

Any changes or follow up needed with medications –

Weight, Blood Pressure, Vitals Reviewed -

POLST reviewed, does patient prefer CPR or DNR?

Upcoming appointments and who will transport –

Insurance/ payer source reviewed –

Anticipated length of stay –

Barriers to address:

Goals: (examples – stitches out, follow up orthopedic appointment for weight bearing upgrade, medication date noted for completion of antibiotic, etc.)

Does the patient have any questions for nursing?

Speech Therapy Review:

Results of any cognitive testing such as the MoCA (Montreal Cognitive Assessment) and what the testing means -

Cognitive strengths noted or deficits –

Swallow Assessment Completed and results –

Any issues noted with swallow –

Diet texture currently –

Any goal to upgrade or downgrade diet texture –

Cognition based recommendations for assistance at home –

Self-medication program recommended or will medication management be recommended?

Physical Therapy Review -

Define what therapy is working on with patient and helping with, strengthening lower body, improving gait, reducing fall risk.

Prior level of function –

Transfer status:

DME used, ie. Hoyer or Mechanical Life, Front wheeled walker, Wheelchair –

Level of assistance needed prior at home/in community –

Level of assistance patient is currently needing, standby assist, contact guard assist, maximum assistance of 2 persons?

Number of feet patient can ambulate –

Does patient use an assistive device such as a front wheeled walker to ambulate or do they self-propel their wheelchair?

Will goal be to return patient as close to prior level of function as possible, or will patient have a new baseline level of function?

Occupational Therapy Review:

Define what occupational therapy is working on with patient and helping with, ie. Activities of daily living or ADL's.

    Prior level of function –

    Amount of assistance needed with lower body dressing –

    Amount of assistance needed with upper body dressing –

    Self Care level of assist, grooming, personal hygiene –

    Level of assistance needed with toileting –

    Transfer status –

    Any recommended adaptive strategies or equipment to promote optimal functioning?

    Recommendation for level of care in community – will increased support be recommended at home or a different setting possibly?

Social Services Review and Discharge Planning:

Discharge Plan:

DME (durable medical equipment) recommended:

Resources and support/caregiver contact info. Given to patient:

Mental Health Services recommended?

Patient accepts or declines mental health interventions: Accepts   Declines

Dental needs:

Vision needs:

Does patient want a Medicaid application and/or help completing?

DPOA established, and if not, does patient need assistance to do so?

Medicare/Insurance Process Reviewed:

Home Health Agency:

Funeral Home selected:

Care Plan Conference   Date:

To identify goals and establish a discharge plan for your rehabilitation patient.

OR Quarterly care conference for long term care resident.

Patient Name: _____

Staff members in attendance names/positions:

Staff Attending Signatures: _____ _____ _____ _____
_____ _____

Family or Friends/ Support Names:

Nursing Review:

Primary diagnosis/ review of recent hospitalization:

- [ ] Copy of Current Care Plan reviewed and provided to patient.
- [ ] Copy of Current Medication List/ Orders reviewed and provided to patient.
- [ ] Does the patient have medication questions?

Any changes or follow up needed with medications –

Weight, Blood Pressure, Vitals Reviewed -

POLST reviewed, does patient prefer CPR or DNR?

Upcoming appointments and who will transport –

Insurance/ payer source reviewed –

Anticipated length of stay –

Barriers to address:

Goals: (examples – stitches out, follow up orthopedic appointment for weight bearing upgrade, medication date noted for completion of antibiotic, etc.)

Does the patient have any questions for nursing?

Speech Therapy Review:

Results of any cognitive testing such as the MoCA (Montreal Cognitive Assessment) and what the testing means -

Cognitive strengths noted or deficits –

Swallow Assessment Completed and results –

Any issues noted with swallow –

Diet texture currently –

Any goal to upgrade or downgrade diet texture –

Cognition based recommendations for assistance at home –

Self-medication program recommended or will medication management be recommended?

Physical Therapy Review -

Define what therapy is working on with patient and helping with, strengthening lower body, improving gait, reducing fall risk.

Prior level of function –

    Transfer status:

    DME used, ie. Hoyer or Mechanical Life, Front wheeled walker, Wheelchair –

    Level of assistance needed prior at home/in community –

    Level of assistance patient is currently needing, standby assist, contact guard assist, maximum assistance of 2 persons?

    Number of feet patient can ambulate –

Does patient use an assistive device such as a front wheeled walker to ambulate or do they self-propel their wheelchair?

    Will goal be to return patient as close to prior level of function as possible, or will patient have a new baseline level of function?

Occupational Therapy Review:

Define what occupational therapy is working on with patient and helping with, ie. Activities of daily living or ADL's.

    Prior level of function –

    Amount of assistance needed with lower body dressing –

    Amount of assistance needed with upper body dressing –

    Self Care level of assist, grooming, personal hygiene –

    Level of assistance needed with toileting –

    Transfer status –

    Any recommended adaptive strategies or equipment to promote optimal functioning?

    Recommendation for level of care in community – will increased support be recommended at home or a different setting possibly?

Social Services Review and Discharge Planning:

Discharge Plan:

DME (durable medical equipment) recommended:

Resources and support/caregiver contact info. Given to patient:

Mental Health Services recommended?

Patient accepts or declines mental health interventions: Accepts   Declines

Dental needs:

Vision needs:

Does patient want a Medicaid application and/or help completing?

DPOA established, and if not, does patient need assistance to do so?

Medicare/Insurance Process Reviewed:

Home Health Agency:

Funeral Home selected:

Care Plan Conference   Date:

To identify goals and establish a discharge plan for your rehabilitation patient.

OR Quarterly care conference for long term care resident.

Patient Name: _____

Staff members in attendance names/positions:

Staff Attending Signatures: _____   _____   _____   _____
_____   _____

Family or Friends/ Support Names:

Nursing Review:

Primary diagnosis/ review of recent hospitalization:

- ➢ Copy of Current Care Plan reviewed and provided to patient.
- ➢ Copy of Current Medication List/ Orders reviewed and provided to patient.
- ➢ Does the patient have medication questions?

Any changes or follow up needed with medications –

Weight, Blood Pressure, Vitals Reviewed -

POLST reviewed, does patient prefer CPR or DNR?

Upcoming appointments and who will transport –

Insurance/ payer source reviewed –

Anticipated length of stay –

Barriers to address:

Goals: (examples – stitches out, follow up orthopedic appointment for weight bearing upgrade, medication date noted for completion of antibiotic, etc.)

Does the patient have any questions for nursing?

Speech Therapy Review:

Results of any cognitive testing such as the MoCA (Montreal Cognitive Assessment) and what the testing means -

Cognitive strengths noted or deficits –

Swallow Assessment Completed and results –

Any issues noted with swallow –

Diet texture currently –

Any goal to upgrade or downgrade diet texture –

Cognition based recommendations for assistance at home –

Self-medication program recommended or will medication management be recommended?

Physical Therapy Review -

Define what therapy is working on with patient and helping with, strengthening lower body, improving gait, reducing fall risk.

Prior level of function –

    Transfer status:

    DME used, ie. Hoyer or Mechanical Life, Front wheeled walker, Wheelchair –

    Level of assistance needed prior at home/in community –

    Level of assistance patient is currently needing, standby assist, contact guard assist, maximum assistance of 2 persons?

Number of feet patient can ambulate –

Does patient use an assistive device such as a front wheeled walker to ambulate or do they self-propel their wheelchair?

Will goal be to return patient as close to prior level of function as possible, or will patient have a new baseline level of function?

Occupational Therapy Review:

Define what occupational therapy is working on with patient and helping with, ie. Activities of daily living or ADL's.

Prior level of function –

Amount of assistance needed with lower body dressing –

Amount of assistance needed with upper body dressing –

Self Care level of assist, grooming, personal hygiene –

Level of assistance needed with toileting –

Transfer status –

Any recommended adaptive strategies or equipment to promote optimal functioning?

Recommendation for level of care in community – will increased support be recommended at home or a different setting possibly?

Social Services Review and Discharge Planning:

Discharge Plan:

DME (durable medical equipment) recommended:

Resources and support/caregiver contact info. Given to patient:

Mental Health Services recommended?

Patient accepts or declines mental health interventions: Accepts   Declines

Dental needs:

Vision needs:

Does patient want a Medicaid application and/or help completing?

DPOA established, and if not, does patient need assistance to do so?

Medicare/Insurance Process Reviewed:

Home Health Agency:

Funeral Home selected:

Care Plan Conference   Date:

To identify goals and establish a discharge plan for your rehabilitation patient.

OR Quarterly care conference for long term care resident.

Patient Name: _____

Staff members in attendance names/positions:

Staff Attending Signatures: _____ _____ _____ _____

_____ _____

Family or Friends/ Support Names:

Nursing Review:

Primary diagnosis/ review of recent hospitalization:

> ➢ Copy of Current Care Plan reviewed and provided to patient.
> ➢ Copy of Current Medication List/ Orders reviewed and provided to

> patient.
> ➢ Does the patient have medication questions?

Any changes or follow up needed with medications –

Weight, Blood Pressure, Vitals Reviewed -

POLST reviewed, does patient prefer CPR or DNR?

Upcoming appointments and who will transport –

Insurance/ payer source reviewed –

Anticipated length of stay –

Barriers to address:

Goals: (examples – stitches out, follow up orthopedic appointment for weight bearing upgrade, medication date noted for completion of antibiotic, etc.)

Does the patient have any questions for nursing?

Speech Therapy Review:

Results of any cognitive testing such as the MoCA (Montreal Cognitive Assessment) and what the testing means -

Cognitive strengths noted or deficits –

Swallow Assessment Completed and results –

Any issues noted with swallow –

Diet texture currently –

Any goal to upgrade or downgrade diet texture –

Cognition based recommendations for assistance at home –

Self-medication program recommended or will medication management be recommended?

Physical Therapy Review -

Define what therapy is working on with patient and helping with, strengthening lower body, improving gait, reducing fall risk.

Prior level of function –

    Transfer status:

DME used, ie. Hoyer or Mechanical Life, Front wheeled walker, Wheelchair –

Level of assistance needed prior at home/in community –

Level of assistance patient is currently needing, standby assist, contact guard assist, maximum assistance of 2 persons?

Number of feet patient can ambulate –

Does patient use an assistive device such as a front wheeled walker to ambulate or do they self-propel their wheelchair?

Will goal be to return patient as close to prior level of function as possible, or will patient have a new baseline level of function?

Occupational Therapy Review:

Define what occupational therapy is working on with patient and helping with, ie. Activities of daily living or ADL's.

Prior level of function –

Amount of assistance needed with lower body dressing –

Amount of assistance needed with upper body dressing –

Self Care level of assist, grooming, personal hygiene –

Level of assistance needed with toileting –

Transfer status –

Any recommended adaptive strategies or equipment to promote optimal functioning?

Recommendation for level of care in community – will increased support be recommended at home or a different setting possibly?

Social Services Review and Discharge Planning:

Discharge Plan:

DME (durable medical equipment) recommended:

Resources and support/caregiver contact info. Given to patient:

Mental Health Services recommended?

Patient accepts or declines mental health interventions: Accepts   Declines

Dental needs:

Vision needs:

Does patient want a Medicaid application and/or help completing?

DPOA established, and if not, does patient need assistance to do so?

Medicare/Insurance Process Reviewed:

Home Health Agency:

Funeral Home selected:

Care Plan Conference   Date:

    To identify goals and establish a discharge plan for your rehabilitation patient.

    OR Quarterly care conference for long term care resident.

Patient Name: _____

Staff members in attendance names/positions:

Staff Attending Signatures: _____   _____   _____   _____
_____   _____

Family or Friends/ Support Names:

Nursing Review:

Primary diagnosis/ review of recent hospitalization:

> ➢ Copy of Current Care Plan reviewed and provided to patient.
> ➢ Copy of Current Medication List/ Orders reviewed and provided to patient.
> ➢ Does the patient have medication questions?

Any changes or follow up needed with medications –

Weight, Blood Pressure, Vitals Reviewed -

POLST reviewed, does patient prefer CPR or DNR?

Upcoming appointments and who will transport –

Insurance/ payer source reviewed –

Anticipated length of stay –

Barriers to address:

Goals: (examples – stitches out, follow up orthopedic appointment for weight bearing upgrade, medication date noted for completion of antibiotic, etc.)

Does the patient have any questions for nursing?

Speech Therapy Review:

Results of any cognitive testing such as the MoCA (Montreal Cognitive Assessment) and what the testing means -

Cognitive strengths noted or deficits –

Swallow Assessment Completed and results –

Any issues noted with swallow –

Diet texture currently –

Any goal to upgrade or downgrade diet texture –

Cognition based recommendations for assistance at home –

Self-medication program recommended or will medication management be recommended?

Physical Therapy Review -

Define what therapy is working on with patient and helping with, strengthening lower body, improving gait, reducing fall risk.

Prior level of function –

    Transfer status:

    DME used, ie. Hoyer or Mechanical Life, Front wheeled walker, Wheelchair –

    Level of assistance needed prior at home/in community –

    Level of assistance patient is currently needing, standby assist, contact guard assist, maximum assistance of 2 persons?

    Number of feet patient can ambulate –

Does patient use an assistive device such as a front wheeled walker to ambulate or do they self-propel their wheelchair?

    Will goal be to return patient as close to prior level of function as possible, or will patient have a new baseline level of function?

Occupational Therapy Review:

Define what occupational therapy is working on with patient and helping with, ie. Activities of daily living or ADL's.

    Prior level of function –

    Amount of assistance needed with lower body dressing –

Amount of assistance needed with upper body dressing –

Self Care level of assist, grooming, personal hygiene –

Level of assistance needed with toileting –

Transfer status –

Any recommended adaptive strategies or equipment to promote optimal functioning?

Recommendation for level of care in community – will increased support be recommended at home or a different setting possibly?

Social Services Review and Discharge Planning:

Discharge Plan:

DME (durable medical equipment) recommended:

Resources and support/caregiver contact info. Given to patient:

Mental Health Services recommended?

Patient accepts or declines mental health interventions: Accepts   Declines

Dental needs:

Vision needs:

Does patient want a Medicaid application and/or help completing?

DPOA established, and if not, does patient need assistance to do so?

Medicare/Insurance Process Reviewed:

Home Health Agency:

Funeral Home selected:

Care Plan Conference   Date:

To identify goals and establish a discharge plan for your rehabilitation patient.

OR Quarterly care conference for long term care resident.

Patient Name: _____

Staff members in attendance names/positions:

Staff Attending Signatures: _____ _____ _____ _____
_____ _____

Family or Friends/ Support Names:

Nursing Review:

Primary diagnosis/ review of recent hospitalization:

- Copy of Current Care Plan reviewed and provided to patient.
- Copy of Current Medication List/ Orders reviewed and provided to patient.
- Does the patient have medication questions?

Any changes or follow up needed with medications –

Weight, Blood Pressure, Vitals Reviewed -

POLST reviewed, does patient prefer CPR or DNR?

Upcoming appointments and who will transport –

Insurance/ payer source reviewed –

Anticipated length of stay –

Barriers to address:

Goals: (examples – stitches out, follow up orthopedic appointment for weight bearing upgrade, medication date noted for completion of antibiotic, etc.)

Does the patient have any questions for nursing?

Speech Therapy Review:

Results of any cognitive testing such as the MoCA (Montreal Cognitive Assessment) and what the testing means -

Cognitive strengths noted or deficits –

Swallow Assessment Completed and results –

Any issues noted with swallow –

Diet texture currently –

Any goal to upgrade or downgrade diet texture –

Cognition based recommendations for assistance at home –

Self-medication program recommended or will medication management be recommended?

Physical Therapy Review -

Define what therapy is working on with patient and helping with, strengthening lower body, improving gait, reducing fall risk.

Prior level of function –

    Transfer status:

    DME used, ie. Hoyer or Mechanical Life, Front wheeled walker, Wheelchair –

    Level of assistance needed prior at home/in community –

    Level of assistance patient is currently needing, standby assist, contact guard assist, maximum assistance of 2 persons?

    Number of feet patient can ambulate –

    Does patient use an assistive device such as a front wheeled walker to ambulate or do they self-propel their wheelchair?

    Will goal be to return patient as close to prior level of function as possible, or will patient have a new baseline level of function?

Occupational Therapy Review:

Define what occupational therapy is working on with patient and helping with, ie. Activities of daily living or ADL's.

    Prior level of function –

    Amount of assistance needed with lower body dressing –

    Amount of assistance needed with upper body dressing –

    Self-Care level of assist, grooming, personal hygiene –

    Level of assistance needed with toileting –

    Transfer status –

    Any recommended adaptive strategies or equipment to promote optimal functioning?

    Recommendation for level of care in community – will increased support be recommended at home or a different setting possibly?

Social Services Review and Discharge Planning:

Discharge Plan:

DME (durable medical equipment) recommended:

Resources and support/caregiver contact info. Given to patient:

Mental Health Services recommended?

Patient accepts or declines mental health interventions: Accepts   Declines

Dental needs:

Vision needs:

Does patient want a Medicaid application and/or help completing?

DPOA established, and if not, does patient need assistance to do so?

Medicare/Insurance Process Reviewed:

Home Health Agency:

Funeral Home selected:

Care Plan Conference   Date:

To identify goals and establish a discharge plan for your rehabilitation patient.

OR Quarterly care conference for long term care resident.

Patient Name: _____

Staff members in attendance names/positions:

Staff Attending Signatures: _____ _____ _____ _____
_____ _____

Family or Friends/ Support Names:

Nursing Review:

Primary diagnosis/ review of recent hospitalization:

- [ ] Copy of Current Care Plan reviewed and provided to patient.
- [ ] Copy of Current Medication List/ Orders reviewed and provided to patient.
- [ ] Does the patient have medication questions?

Any changes or follow up needed with medications –

Weight, Blood Pressure, Vitals Reviewed -

POLST reviewed, does patient prefer CPR or DNR?

Upcoming appointments and who will transport –

Insurance/ payer source reviewed –

Anticipated length of stay –

Barriers to address:

Goals: (examples – stitches out, follow up orthopedic appointment for weight bearing upgrade, medication date noted for completion of antibiotic, etc.)

Does the patient have any questions for nursing?

Speech Therapy Review:

Results of any cognitive testing such as the MoCA (Montreal Cognitive Assessment) and what the testing means -

Cognitive strengths noted or deficits –

Swallow Assessment Completed and results –

Any issues noted with swallow –

Diet texture currently –

Any goal to upgrade or downgrade diet texture –

Cognition based recommendations for assistance at home –

Self-medication program recommended or will medication management be recommended?

Physical Therapy Review -

Define what therapy is working on with patient and helping with, strengthening lower body, improving gait, reducing fall risk.

Prior level of function –

    Transfer status:

    DME used, ie. Hoyer or Mechanical Life, Front wheeled walker, Wheelchair –

    Level of assistance needed prior at home/in community –

    Level of assistance patient is currently needing, standby assist, contact guard assist, maximum assistance of 2 persons?

    Number of feet patient can ambulate –

    Does patient use an assistive device such as a front wheeled walker to ambulate or do they self-propel their wheelchair?

    Will goal be to return patient as close to prior level of function as possible, or will patient have a new baseline level of function?

Occupational Therapy Review:

Define what occupational therapy is working on with patient and helping with, ie. Activities of daily living or ADL's.

    Prior level of function –

    Amount of assistance needed with lower body dressing –

    Amount of assistance needed with upper body dressing –

    Self Care level of assist, grooming, personal hygiene –

    Level of assistance needed with toileting –

    Transfer status –

    Any recommended adaptive strategies or equipment to promote optimal functioning?

    Recommendation for level of care in community – will increased support be recommended at home or a different setting possibly?

Social Services Review and Discharge Planning:

Discharge Plan:

DME (durable medical equipment) recommended:

Resources and support/caregiver contact info. Given to patient:

Mental Health Services recommended?

Patient accepts or declines mental health interventions: Accepts   Declines

Dental needs:

Vision needs:

Does patient want a Medicaid application and/or help completing?

DPOA established, and if not, does patient need assistance to do so?

Medicare/Insurance Process Reviewed:

Home Health Agency:

Funeral Home selected:

Care Plan Conference   Date:

To identify goals and establish a discharge plan for your rehabilitation patient.

OR Quarterly care conference for long term care resident.

Patient Name: _____

Staff members in attendance names/positions:

Staff Attending Signatures: _____ _____ _____ _____

_____ _____

Family or Friends/ Support Names:

Nursing Review:

Primary diagnosis/ review of recent hospitalization:

- Copy of Current Care Plan reviewed and provided to patient.
- Copy of Current Medication List/ Orders reviewed and provided to patient.
- Does the patient have medication questions?

Any changes or follow up needed with medications –

Weight, Blood Pressure, Vitals Reviewed -

POLST reviewed, does patient prefer CPR or DNR?

Upcoming appointments and who will transport –

Insurance/ payer source reviewed –

Anticipated length of stay –

Barriers to address:

Goals: (examples – stitches out, follow up orthopedic appointment for weight bearing upgrade, medication date noted for completion of antibiotic, etc.)

Does the patient have any questions for nursing?

Speech Therapy Review:

Results of any cognitive testing such as the MoCA (Montreal Cognitive Assessment) and what the testing means -

Cognitive strengths noted or deficits –

Swallow Assessment Completed and results –

Any issues noted with swallow –

Diet texture currently –

Any goal to upgrade or downgrade diet texture –

Cognition based recommendations for assistance at home –

Self-medication program recommended or will medication management be recommended?

Physical Therapy Review -

Define what therapy is working on with patient and helping with, strengthening lower body, improving gait, reducing fall risk.

Prior level of function –

    Transfer status:

    DME used, ie. Hoyer or Mechanical Life, Front wheeled walker, Wheelchair –

    Level of assistance needed prior at home/in community –

    Level of assistance patient is currently needing, standby assist, contact guard assist, maximum assistance of 2 persons?

    Number of feet patient can ambulate –

Does patient use an assistive device such as a front wheeled walker to ambulate or do they self-propel their wheelchair?

Will goal be to return patient as close to prior level of function as possible, or will patient have a new baseline level of function?

Occupational Therapy Review:

Define what occupational therapy is working on with patient and helping with, ie. Activities of daily living or ADL's.

Prior level of function –

Amount of assistance needed with lower body dressing –

Amount of assistance needed with upper body dressing –

Self Care level of assist, grooming, personal hygiene –

Level of assistance needed with toileting –

Transfer status –

Any recommended adaptive strategies or equipment to promote optimal functioning?

Recommendation for level of care in community – will increased support be recommended at home or a different setting possibly?

Social Services Review and Discharge Planning:

Discharge Plan:

DME (durable medical equipment) recommended:

Resources and support/caregiver contact info. Given to patient:

Mental Health Services recommended?

Patient accepts or declines mental health interventions: Accepts   Declines

Dental needs:

Vision needs:

Does patient want a Medicaid application and/or help completing?

DPOA established, and if not, does patient need assistance to do so?

Medicare/Insurance Process Reviewed:

Home Health Agency:

Funeral Home selected:

Care Plan Conference   Date:

To identify goals and establish a discharge plan for your rehabilitation patient.

OR Quarterly care conference for long term care resident.

Patient Name: _____

Staff members in attendance names/positions:

Staff Attending Signatures: _____ _____ _____ _____

_____ _____

Family or Friends/ Support Names:

Nursing Review:

Primary diagnosis/ review of recent hospitalization:

   ➢ Copy of Current Care Plan reviewed and provided to patient.
   ➢ Copy of Current Medication List/ Orders reviewed and provided to

patient.
➢ Does the patient have medication questions?

Any changes or follow up needed with medications –

Weight, Blood Pressure, Vitals Reviewed -

POLST reviewed, does patient prefer CPR or DNR?

Upcoming appointments and who will transport –

Insurance/ payer source reviewed –

Anticipated length of stay –

Barriers to address:

Goals: (examples – stitches out, follow up orthopedic appointment for weight bearing upgrade, medication date noted for completion of antibiotic, etc.)

Does the patient have any questions for nursing?

Speech Therapy Review:

Results of any cognitive testing such as the MoCA (Montreal Cognitive Assessment) and what the testing means -

Cognitive strengths noted or deficits –

Swallow Assessment Completed and results –

Any issues noted with swallow –

Diet texture currently –

Any goal to upgrade or downgrade diet texture –

Cognition based recommendations for assistance at home –

Self-medication program recommended or will medication management be recommended?

Physical Therapy Review -

Define what therapy is working on with patient and helping with, strengthening lower body, improving gait, reducing fall risk.

Prior level of function –

    Transfer status:

    DME used, ie. Hoyer or Mechanical Life, Front wheeled walker, Wheelchair –

Level of assistance needed prior at home/in community –

Level of assistance patient is currently needing, standby assist, contact guard assist, maximum assistance of 2 persons?

Number of feet patient can ambulate –

Does patient use an assistive device such as a front wheeled walker to ambulate or do they self-propel their wheelchair?

Will goal be to return patient as close to prior level of function as possible, or will patient have a new baseline level of function?

Occupational Therapy Review:

Define what occupational therapy is working on with patient and helping with, ie. Activities of daily living or ADL's.

Prior level of function –

Amount of assistance needed with lower body dressing –

Amount of assistance needed with upper body dressing –

Self Care level of assist, grooming, personal hygiene –

Level of assistance needed with toileting –

Transfer status –

Any recommended adaptive strategies or equipment to promote optimal functioning?

Recommendation for level of care in community – will increased support be recommended at home or a different setting possibly?

Social Services Review and Discharge Planning:

Discharge Plan:

DME (durable medical equipment) recommended:

Resources and support/caregiver contact info. Given to patient:

Mental Health Services recommended?

Patient accepts or declines mental health interventions: Accepts   Declines

Dental needs:

Vision needs:

Does patient want a Medicaid application and/or help completing?

DPOA established, and if not, does patient need assistance to do so?

Medicare/Insurance Process Reviewed:

Home Health Agency:

Funeral Home selected:

Care Plan Conference   Date:

To identify goals and establish a discharge plan for your rehabilitation patient.

OR Quarterly care conference for long term care resident.

Patient Name: _____

Staff members in attendance names/positions:

Staff Attending Signatures: _____ _____ _____ _____

_____ _____

Family or Friends/ Support Names:

Nursing Review:

Primary diagnosis/ review of recent hospitalization:

- Copy of Current Care Plan reviewed and provided to patient.
- Copy of Current Medication List/ Orders reviewed and provided to patient.
- Does the patient have medication questions?

Any changes or follow up needed with medications –

Weight, Blood Pressure, Vitals Reviewed -

POLST reviewed, does patient prefer CPR or DNR?

Upcoming appointments and who will transport –

Insurance/ payer source reviewed –

Anticipated length of stay –

Barriers to address:

Goals: (examples – stitches out, follow up orthopedic appointment for weight bearing upgrade, medication date noted for completion of antibiotic, etc.)

Does the patient have any questions for nursing?

Speech Therapy Review:

Results of any cognitive testing such as the MoCA (Montreal Cognitive Assessment) and what the testing means -

Cognitive strengths noted or deficits –

Swallow Assessment Completed and results –

Any issues noted with swallow –

Diet texture currently –

Any goal to upgrade or downgrade diet texture –

Cognition based recommendations for assistance at home –

Self-medication program recommended or will medication management be recommended?

Physical Therapy Review -

Define what therapy is working on with patient and helping with, strengthening lower body, improving gait, reducing fall risk.

Prior level of function –

    Transfer status:

    DME used, ie. Hoyer or Mechanical Life, Front wheeled walker, Wheelchair –

    Level of assistance needed prior at home/in community –

    Level of assistance patient is currently needing, standby assist, contact guard assist, maximum assistance of 2 persons?

    Number of feet patient can ambulate –

Does patient use an assistive device such as a front wheeled walker to ambulate or do they self-propel their wheelchair?

    Will goal be to return patient as close to prior level of function as possible, or will patient have a new baseline level of function?

Occupational Therapy Review:

Define what occupational therapy is working on with patient and helping with, ie. Activities of daily living or ADL's.

    Prior level of function –

    Amount of assistance needed with lower body dressing –

Amount of assistance needed with upper body dressing –

Self Care level of assist, grooming, personal hygiene –

Level of assistance needed with toileting –

Transfer status –

Any recommended adaptive strategies or equipment to promote optimal functioning?

Recommendation for level of care in community – will increased support be recommended at home or a different setting possibly?

Social Services Review and Discharge Planning:

Discharge Plan:

DME (durable medical equipment) recommended:

Resources and support/caregiver contact info. Given to patient:

Mental Health Services recommended?

Patient accepts or declines mental health interventions: Accepts   Declines

Dental needs:

Vision needs:

Does patient want a Medicaid application and/or help completing?

DPOA established, and if not, does patient need assistance to do so?

Medicare/Insurance Process Reviewed:

Home Health Agency:

Funeral Home selected:

Care Plan Conference Date:

    To identify goals and establish a discharge plan for your rehabilitation patient.

    OR Quarterly care conference for long term care resident.

Patient Name: _____

Staff members in attendance names/positions:

Staff Attending Signatures: _____ _____ _____ _____
_____ _____

Family or Friends/ Support Names:

Nursing Review:

Primary diagnosis/ review of recent hospitalization:

- ➤ Copy of Current Care Plan reviewed and provided to patient.
- ➤ Copy of Current Medication List/ Orders reviewed and provided to patient.
- ➤ Does the patient have medication questions?

Any changes or follow up needed with medications –

Weight, Blood Pressure, Vitals Reviewed -

POLST reviewed, does patient prefer CPR or DNR?

Upcoming appointments and who will transport –

Insurance/ payer source reviewed –

Anticipated length of stay –

Barriers to address:

Goals: (examples – stitches out, follow up orthopedic appointment for weight bearing upgrade, medication date noted for completion of antibiotic, etc.)

Does the patient have any questions for nursing?

Speech Therapy Review:

Results of any cognitive testing such as the MoCA (Montreal Cognitive Assessment) and what the testing means -

Cognitive strengths noted or deficits –

Swallow Assessment Completed and results –

Any issues noted with swallow –

Diet texture currently –

Any goal to upgrade or downgrade diet texture –

Cognition based recommendations for assistance at home –

Self-medication program recommended or will medication management be recommended?

Physical Therapy Review -

Define what therapy is working on with patient and helping with, strengthening lower body, improving gait, reducing fall risk.

Prior level of function –

    Transfer status:

    DME used, ie. Hoyer or Mechanical Life, Front wheeled walker, Wheelchair –

    Level of assistance needed prior at home/in community –

    Level of assistance patient is currently needing, standby assist, contact guard assist, maximum assistance of 2 persons?

    Number of feet patient can ambulate –

Does patient use an assistive device such as a front wheeled walker to ambulate or do they self-propel their wheelchair?

    Will goal be to return patient as close to prior level of function as possible, or will patient have a new baseline level of function?

Occupational Therapy Review:

Define what occupational therapy is working on with patient and helping with, ie. Activities of daily living or ADL's.

Prior level of function –

Amount of assistance needed with lower body dressing –

Amount of assistance needed with upper body dressing –

Self Care level of assist, grooming, personal hygiene –

Level of assistance needed with toileting –

Transfer status –

Any recommended adaptive strategies or equipment to promote optimal functioning?

Recommendation for level of care in community – will increased support be recommended at home or a different setting possibly?

Social Services Review and Discharge Planning:

Discharge Plan:

DME (durable medical equipment) recommended:

Resources and support/caregiver contact info. Given to patient:

Mental Health Services recommended?

Patient accepts or declines mental health interventions: Accepts   Declines

Dental needs:

Vision needs:

Does patient want a Medicaid application and/or help completing?

DPOA established, and if not, does patient need assistance to do so?

Medicare/Insurance Process Reviewed:

Home Health Agency:

Funeral Home selected:

Care Plan Conference   Date:

    To identify goals and establish a discharge plan for your rehabilitation patient.

OR Quarterly care conference for long term care resident.

Patient Name: _____

Staff members in attendance names/positions:

Staff Attending Signatures: _____ _____ _____ _____
_____ _____

Family or Friends/ Support Names:

Nursing Review:

Primary diagnosis/ review of recent hospitalization:

- ➢ Copy of Current Care Plan reviewed and provided to patient.
- ➢ Copy of Current Medication List/ Orders reviewed and provided to patient.
- ➢ Does the patient have medication questions?

Any changes or follow up needed with medications –

Weight, Blood Pressure, Vitals Reviewed -

POLST reviewed, does patient prefer CPR or DNR?

Upcoming appointments and who will transport –

Insurance/ payer source reviewed –

Anticipated length of stay –

Barriers to address:

Goals: (examples – stitches out, follow up orthopedic appointment for weight bearing upgrade, medication date noted for completion of antibiotic, etc.)

Does the patient have any questions for nursing?

Speech Therapy Review:

Results of any cognitive testing such as the MoCA (Montreal Cognitive Assessment) and what the testing means -

Cognitive strengths noted or deficits –

Swallow Assessment Completed and results –

Any issues noted with swallow –

Diet texture currently –

Any goal to upgrade or downgrade diet texture –

Cognition based recommendations for assistance at home –

Self-medication program recommended or will medication management be recommended?

Physical Therapy Review -

Define what therapy is working on with patient and helping with, strengthening lower body, improving gait, reducing fall risk.

Prior level of function –

    Transfer status:

    DME used, ie. Hoyer or Mechanical Life, Front wheeled walker, Wheelchair –

    Level of assistance needed prior at home/in community –

    Level of assistance patient is currently needing, standby assist, contact guard assist, maximum assistance of 2 persons?

    Number of feet patient can ambulate –

    Does patient use an assistive device such as a front wheeled walker to ambulate or do they self-propel their wheelchair?

    Will goal be to return patient as close to prior level of function as possible, or will patient have a new baseline level of function?

Occupational Therapy Review:

Define what occupational therapy is working on with patient and helping with, ie. Activities of daily living or ADL's.

    Prior level of function –

    Amount of assistance needed with lower body dressing –

    Amount of assistance needed with upper body dressing –

    Self-Care level of assist, grooming, personal hygiene –

    Level of assistance needed with toileting –

    Transfer status –

    Any recommended adaptive strategies or equipment to promote optimal functioning?

    Recommendation for level of care in community – will increased support be recommended at home or a different setting possibly?

Social Services Review and Discharge Planning:

Discharge Plan:

DME (durable medical equipment) recommended:

Resources and support/caregiver contact info. Given to patient:

Mental Health Services recommended?

Patient accepts or declines mental health interventions: Accepts   Declines

Dental needs:

Vision needs:

Does patient want a Medicaid application and/or help completing?

DPOA established, and if not, does patient need assistance to do so?

Medicare/Insurance Process Reviewed:

Home Health Agency:

Funeral Home selected:

Care Plan Conference   Date:

To identify goals and establish a discharge plan for your rehabilitation patient.

OR Quarterly care conference for long term care resident.

Patient Name: _____

Staff members in attendance names/positions:

Staff Attending Signatures: _____ _____ _____ _____
_____ _____

Family or Friends/ Support Names:

Nursing Review:

Primary diagnosis/ review of recent hospitalization:

- [ ] Copy of Current Care Plan reviewed and provided to patient.
- [ ] Copy of Current Medication List/ Orders reviewed and provided to patient.
- [ ] Does the patient have medication questions?

Any changes or follow up needed with medications –

Weight, Blood Pressure, Vitals Reviewed -

POLST reviewed, does patient prefer CPR or DNR?

Upcoming appointments and who will transport –

Insurance/ payer source reviewed –

Anticipated length of stay –

Barriers to address:

Goals: (examples – stitches out, follow up orthopedic appointment for weight bearing upgrade, medication date noted for completion of antibiotic, etc.)

Does the patient have any questions for nursing?

Speech Therapy Review:

Results of any cognitive testing such as the MoCA (Montreal Cognitive Assessment) and what the testing means -

Cognitive strengths noted or deficits –

Swallow Assessment Completed and results –

Any issues noted with swallow –

Diet texture currently –

Any goal to upgrade or downgrade diet texture –

Cognition based recommendations for assistance at home –

Self-medication program recommended or will medication management be recommended?

Physical Therapy Review -

Define what therapy is working on with patient and helping with, strengthening lower body, improving gait, reducing fall risk.

Prior level of function –

    Transfer status:

    DME used, ie. Hoyer or Mechanical Life, Front wheeled walker, Wheelchair –

    Level of assistance needed prior at home/in community –

    Level of assistance patient is currently needing, standby assist, contact guard assist, maximum assistance of 2 persons?

    Number of feet patient can ambulate –

    Does patient use an assistive device such as a front wheeled walker to ambulate or do they self-propel their wheelchair?

Will goal be to return patient as close to prior level of function as possible, or will patient have a new baseline level of function?

Occupational Therapy Review:

Define what occupational therapy is working on with patient and helping with, ie. Activities of daily living or ADL's.

Prior level of function –

Amount of assistance needed with lower body dressing –

Amount of assistance needed with upper body dressing –

Self Care level of assist, grooming, personal hygiene –

Level of assistance needed with toileting –

Transfer status –

Any recommended adaptive strategies or equipment to promote optimal functioning?

Recommendation for level of care in community – will increased support be recommended at home or a different setting possibly?

Social Services Review and Discharge Planning:

Discharge Plan:

DME (durable medical equipment) recommended:

Resources and support/caregiver contact info. Given to patient:

Mental Health Services recommended?

Patient accepts or declines mental health interventions: Accepts   Declines

Dental needs:

Vision needs:

Does patient want a Medicaid application and/or help completing?

DPOA established, and if not, does patient need assistance to do so?

Medicare/Insurance Process Reviewed:

Home Health Agency:

Funeral Home selected:

Care Plan Conference   Date:

To identify goals and establish a discharge plan for your rehabilitation patient.

OR Quarterly care conference for long term care resident.

Patient Name: _____

Staff members in attendance names/positions:

Staff Attending Signatures: _____ _____ _____ _____

_____ _____

Family or Friends/ Support Names:

Nursing Review:

Primary diagnosis/ review of recent hospitalization:

- ☐ Copy of Current Care Plan reviewed and provided to patient.
- ☐ Copy of Current Medication List/ Orders reviewed and provided to patient.
- ☐ Does the patient have medication questions?

Any changes or follow up needed with medications –

Weight, Blood Pressure, Vitals Reviewed -

POLST reviewed, does patient prefer CPR or DNR?

Upcoming appointments and who will transport –

Insurance/ payer source reviewed –

Anticipated length of stay –

Barriers to address:

Goals: (examples – stitches out, follow up orthopedic appointment for weight bearing upgrade, medication date noted for completion of antibiotic, etc.)

Does the patient have any questions for nursing?

Speech Therapy Review:

Results of any cognitive testing such as the MoCA (Montreal Cognitive Assessment) and what the testing means -

Cognitive strengths noted or deficits –

Swallow Assessment Completed and results –

Any issues noted with swallow –

Diet texture currently –

Any goal to upgrade or downgrade diet texture –

Cognition based recommendations for assistance at home –

Self-medication program recommended or will medication management be recommended?

Physical Therapy Review -

Define what therapy is working on with patient and helping with, strengthening lower body, improving gait, reducing fall risk.

Prior level of function –

    Transfer status:

    DME used, ie. Hoyer or Mechanical Life, Front wheeled walker, Wheelchair –

    Level of assistance needed prior at home/in community –

Level of assistance patient is currently needing, standby assist, contact guard assist, maximum assistance of 2 persons?

Number of feet patient can ambulate –

Does patient use an assistive device such as a front wheeled walker to ambulate or do they self-propel their wheelchair?

Will goal be to return patient as close to prior level of function as possible, or will patient have a new baseline level of function?

Occupational Therapy Review:

Define what occupational therapy is working on with patient and helping with, ie. Activities of daily living or ADL's.

Prior level of function –

Amount of assistance needed with lower body dressing –

Amount of assistance needed with upper body dressing –

Self Care level of assist, grooming, personal hygiene –

Level of assistance needed with toileting –

Transfer status –

Any recommended adaptive strategies or equipment to promote optimal functioning?

Recommendation for level of care in community – will increased support be recommended at home or a different setting possibly?

Social Services Review and Discharge Planning:

Discharge Plan:

DME (durable medical equipment) recommended:

Resources and support/caregiver contact info. Given to patient:

Mental Health Services recommended?

Patient accepts or declines mental health interventions: Accepts   Declines

Dental needs:

Vision needs:

Does patient want a Medicaid application and/or help completing?

DPOA established, and if not, does patient need assistance to do so?

Medicare/Insurance Process Reviewed:

Home Health Agency:

Funeral Home selected:

www.ingramcontent.com/pod-product-compliance
Lightning Source LLC
Chambersburg PA
CBHW080513220526
45465CB00006B/2469